Prentice Hall Health's

Survival Guide

FOR

LONG-TERM CARE

NURSING ASSISTANTS

Marti Burton, RN, BS
Health Education Curriculum Developer
for the Oklahoma Department of Career
and Technology Education

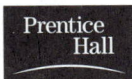

Prentice
Hall

Upper Saddle River, New Jersey 07458

Publisher: Julie Alexander
Executive Editor: Maura Connor
Acquisitions Editor: Barbara Krawiec
Director of Production and Manufacturing: Bruce Johnson
Managing Production Editor: Patrick Walsh
Production Editor: Jeanne Lewis Grogan, Navta Associates, Inc.
Production Liaison: Danielle Newhouse
Manufacturing Manager: Ilene Sanford
Creative Director: Marianne Frasco
Cover Design Coordinator: Maria Guglielmo
Cover Designer: Joseph Sengotta
Marketing Manager: David Hough
Marketing Coordinator: Rachele Triano
Editorial Assistant: Melissa Kerian
Composition: Navta Associates, Inc.
Printing and Binding: The Banta Company

Prentice-Hall International (UK) Limited, *London*
Prentice-Hall of Australia Pty. Limited, *Sydney*
Prentice-Hall Canada Inc., *Toronto*
Prentice-Hall Hispanoamericana, S.A., *Mexico*
Prentice-Hall of India Private Limited, *New Delhi*
Prentice-Hall of Japan, Inc., *Tokyo*
Prentice-Hall Singapore Pte. Ltd.
Editora Prentice-Hall do Brasil, Ltda., *Rio de Janeiro*

Prentice
Hall

10 9 8 7 6 5 4
ISBN 0-13-092067-3

CONTENTS

PREFACE

The thirteen topics in this booklet were selected to provide quick, clear guidance to nursing assistants working in long-term care. The guide includes key points in providing care for residents with respiratory problems, circulatory problems, stroke, and diabetes. Because new graduates of nursing assistant courses often find it difficult to remember medical terminology, abbreviations, and the normal ranges of vital signs, these are included. This survival guide provides a quick way to look up what the nursing assistant does not remember or has not yet applied. The booklet also contains key points about observing, reporting, recording, and identifying abnormals. These sections help the nursing assistant focus on finding abnormals and reporting them immediately. The final topic of the booklet provides key information to help nursing assistants be prepared for state survey team visits. It is my hope that nursing assistants in long-term care will feel more confident with this survival guide in their pockets. It is also my hope that they will give quality care as a result of their confidence and these guidelines.

Reviewers

Dr. Sheila Guidry, RN
Wallace Community College
Selma, AL

Julie Capriola, RN
Coordinator of the Nurses
    Aide Program
Vance Granville Community
    College
Henderson, NC

Joan Scribner, RN, BSN
Affiliate Faculty
Metropolitan Community
    College
Kansas City, MO

Barbara Magerl, RN,
    BSN, MS
Executive Director
Horizon Career College
Merrillville, IN

Acknowledgments

I would like to thank Barbara Krawiec at Prentice Hall for believing that I could write a book, even when I wasn't convinced. And I would like to thank my family for their love and support in all my writing endeavors.

Notice

The procedures described in this textbook are based on consultation with nursing authorities. The author and publisher have taken care to make certain that these procedures reflect currently accepted clinical practice; however, they cannot be considered absolute recommendations.

The material in this textbook contains the most current information available at the time of publication. However, federal, state and local guidelines concerning clinical practices, including without limitation, those governing infection control and universal precautions, change rapidly. The reader should note, therefore, that new regulations may require changes in some procedures.

It is the responsibility of the reader to familiarize himself or herself with the policies and procedures set by federal, state and local agencies, as well as the institution or agency where the reader is employed. The authors and the publishers of this textbook, and the supplements written to accompany it, disclaim any liability, loss or risk resulting directly or indirectly from the suggested procedures and theory, from any undetected errors, or from the reader's misunderstanding of the text. It is the reader's responsibility to stay informed of any new changes or recommendations made by any federal, state and local agency as well as by his or her employing health care institution or agency.

1 MASTERING MEDICAL TERMINOLOGY

Health care has a language of its own. Medical terminology and abbreviations are used to communicate with nursing care staff, physicians, and other health care workers. Many medical terms can be separated into prefixes, root words, and suffixes. When you know the meaning of each part of the word, you can "translate" the meaning of the whole word. Abbreviations are a form of shorthand for quickly writing about patient care. It is important for you to understand medical terminology and abbreviations to communicate effectively with other health care workers. Here are some tips to help you master medical terminology.

Reviewing Root Words

♦ The root word provides the basic meaning of a word. Some frequently used root words and their meanings are:

arthro = joint
cardio = heart
colo   = colon
derma = skin
gastro = stomach
glyco = sugar
hema   = blood
myo   = muscle
neuro = nerve

```
osteo   = bone
psycho = mind
pulmo  = lung
```

♦ Break a word apart to find its meaning. Determine the meaning of the root word first, then move to the prefix and/or suffix.

♦ Look up root words that you do not know and do not find in the list. Use a medical dictionary or long-term care nursing assistant textbook to find the meaning of the root word.

Remembering Prefixes

♦ Prefixes come before a root word. A prefix combines with a root word to form a new word. Some commonly used prefixes and their meanings are:

```
a-, an- = without, not
ab-     = away from
ad-     = toward
ante-   = before
anti-   = against
bi-     = double, or two
brady-  = slow
dys-    = difficult, abnormal
hemi-   = half
hyper-  = above normal, high
hypo-   = below normal, low
post-   = after, behind
pre-    = before, in front
tachy-  = fast
```

♦ Look up prefixes that you do not know and do not find in the list. Use a medical dictionary or other reference book to find the meaning.

Solving Suffixes

♦ Suffixes come after a root word. A suffix combines with a root word to form a new word. Some common suffixes and their meanings are:

-algia   = pain
-ectomy = surgical removal
-emia   = in the blood
-itis   = inflammation of
-ology = study of
-ostomy = surgically created opening
-opathy = disease
-phasia = speaking
-phobia = fear
-plegia = paralysis
-pnea   = to breathe
-uria   = urine

♦ Look up suffixes that you do not know and do not find in the list. Use a medical dictionary or long-term care nursing assistant textbook to find the meaning.

Translating Abbreviations

♦ Abbreviations may use the first letter of each word they represent or the first and last letter of a word.

- ◆ Abbreviations may use the first three or four letters of a word or use a chemical symbol to represent the word.

- ◆ Some common medical abbreviations and their meanings are:

ac	=	before meals
ADLs	=	activities of daily living
ad lib	=	as desired
A.M.	=	morning
amb	=	ambulate
bid	=	twice a day
BM	=	bowel movement
BP	=	blood pressure
BR	=	bathroom
BRP	=	bathroom privileges
BSC	=	bedside commode
c̄	=	with
c/o	=	complains of
CVA	=	cerebrovascular accident or stroke
dc	=	discontinue or discharge
DON	=	director of nurses
GI	=	gastrointestinal
HOH	=	hard of hearing
hr, h	=	hour
HS	=	hour of sleep or bedtime
I&O	=	intake and output
IV	=	intravenous
meds	=	medications

NPO = nothing by mouth
02 = oxygen
OOB = out of bed
$\bar{p}$ = after
pc = after meals
P.M. = afternoon
po = by mouth
prn = when necessary/as needed
pt = patient
$\bar{q}$ = every
qam = every morning
qh = every hour
qhs = every night at bedtime
qid = four times a day
qod = every other day
ROM = range of motion
$\bar{s}$ = without
SOB = short of breath
stat = immediately or at once
tid = three times a day
TLC = tender loving care
TPR = temperature, pulse, and respiration
VS = vital signs
w/c = wheelchair
wt = weight

♦ Use only standard abbreviations when communicating with other health care workers or writing on a resident's chart.

Using appropriate precautions for preventing the spread of infection is vital for the residents' health and your own. You will use standard precautions every day. Some types of precautions may be used only rarely, depending on the residents' needs. To be safe, you need to be sure. Some guidelines to help you are:

♦ Standard Precautions are used with all residents to prevent contact with blood and body fluids, which could cause infection in the health care worker.

Handwashing

♦ Wash your hands immediately after any accidental contact with blood, body fluids, secretions, open skin, or mucous membranes.

♦ Wash your hands every time you put on gloves and every time you take gloves off.

Using Personal Protective Equipment

♦ Wear gloves whenever you give direct care or anytime there is a risk of touching blood, body fluids, secretions, open skin, or mucous membranes.

♦ Wear a gown if there is a chance your clothing could come in contact with any of these substances.

♦ Wear a mask, goggles, or face shield when there is a chance of blood, body fluids, or secretions being splashed or otherwise coming in contact with your face, mouth, or eyes.

Handling Used Equipment and Supplies

♦ Treat all soiled linens and trash as infectious material.

♦ Dispose of used sharp objects such as needles and lancets in the proper sharps container.

♦ Clean and disinfect all reusable equipment according to the policy of the long-term care facility.

3 TAKING CHARGE OF TRANSMISSION-BASED PRECAUTIONS

The use of transmission-based precautions is to prevent the spread of a communicable disease from an infected resident to other residents and to staff. Transmission-based precautions vary depending on the type of infection that exists. Below is a quick reference for using transmission-based precautions.

♦ Always use standard precautions in addition to these transmission-based precautions.

Using Contact Precautions

♦ Contact precautions are used to prevent infection from spreading through contact with the infected person or through contact with surfaces or items that could be contaminated by the infected person. Some examples of infections requiring contact precautions are:

wound infections such as staph infections and methicillin-resistant Staph aureus (MRSA)

intestinal infections that cause symptoms such as vomiting and diarrhea

hepatitis A (spread by contact with feces or saliva of infected person)

♦ When you care for a resident on contact precautions, you should:

wear gloves for all contact with the resident and the resident's items wear a gown if your clothes will have contact with the resident or contaminated items

wear a mask and eyewear if there is a chance of the infectious organism coming in contact with your face, mouth, or eyes

wash your hands after removing your gloves, being careful not to touch any surfaces or items in the resident's room

instruct visitors to report to the nurses' station before entering the room

Using Droplet Precautions

♦ Droplet precautions are used to prevent infection from spreading in droplets of moisture that are exhaled when the resident talks, coughs, or sneezes. Some examples of infections spread by droplets are:

pneumonia

strep throat

common cold

♦ When you care for a resident on droplet precautions, you should:

wear a mask when entering the resident's room or when working within 3 feet of the resident

wear gloves according to standard precautions

wear a gown according to standard precautions

wash your hands before and after wearing gloves

put a mask on the resident if he or she must leave the room

clean and disinfect any equipment used on this resident before using it for other residents

instruct visitors to report to the nurses' station before entering the room

Using Airborne Precautions

♦ Airborne precautions are used to prevent infection from spreading through small droplets in the air that could be inhaled by staff or other residents. Some examples of infections spread by the airborne route are:

tuberculosis

shingles

♦ When you care for a resident on airborne precautions, you should

wear a respirator for residents with known or suspected tuberculosis

wear a standard mask for other diseases

keep the doors to the room closed at all times

wash your hands before and after wearing gloves

wear gloves according to standard precautions

wear a gown according to standard precautions

clean and disinfect any equipment used on this resident before using it for other residents

instruct visitors to report to the nurses' station before entering the room

4 BEING VICTORIOUS OVER VITAL SIGN ERRORS

When you measure a resident's vital signs, accuracy is extremely important. Remember to take your time during the procedures and be sure of your findings. Ask for help if you are unsure of your results. Some additional tips for vanquishing vital sign errors are:

♦ Vital signs include temperature, pulse, respiration, and blood pressure. Include all of these when you are requested to take a resident's vital signs.

♦ You may be requested to take a resident's "TPR." This means to take a full set of vital signs unless you are instructed differently.

Measuring the Temperature

♦ Normal temperatures vary depending on the route used for obtaining the measurement.

Oral temperature	98.6° F
Rectal temperature	99.6° F
Axillary temperature	97.6° F
Tympanic temperature	98.6° F

♦ Delay taking an oral temperature until 15 minutes after the resident has had anything to eat or drink.

♦ When taking a rectal temperature, use a red-topped thermometer. Always lubricate the tip or use a prelubricated sheath.

♦ Check glass thermometers for chips, cracks, or breaks before using them. Dispose of a damaged thermometer according to facility guidelines.

Counting the Pulse and Respirations

♦ Count the radial pulse on the thumb-side of the inner wrist. Count the beats you feel for a full minute if the pulse is irregular; count the beats for 30 seconds and multiply the number by two for a regular pulse.

♦ Count the respirations immediately after counting the pulse, without the resident's awareness. One rise *and* fall of the chest equals one respiration. Count for 30 seconds and multiply the number by two; count for a full minute if the respirations are irregular.

♦ Normal pulse and respiration ranges are:

Pulse   60 to 90 beats per minute
Respirations   16 to 20 breaths per minute

Measuring Blood Pressure

♦ Wrap the blood pressure cuff (sphygmomanometer) around the resident's arm so the bottom edge is one inch above the elbow. Position it so the arrow on the cuff is pointing to the resident's brachial artery.

♦ Tighten the valve on the cuff by turning it to the right. Loosen it by turning it to the left.

♦ Listen carefully for the first beat and the last beat you hear. Remember both numbers until you can write them down.

♦ Release all the air from the cuff by turning the valve completely to the left.

♦ If you are not sure of the reading, completely deflate the cuff. Let the resident's arm rest for at least one minute before you reinflate the cuff again.

♦ Normal blood pressure ranges are:

Systolic (top number measured during heart beat)	100 to 140 mm Hg
Diastolic (bottom number measured when heart is at rest)	60 to 90 mm Hg

♦ Take blood pressure only in an arm that does not have an IV, a dialysis shunt, a wound, or a sore present.

As a certified nursing assistant, you will communicate with residents, their families and friends, and coworkers. Sometimes you will communicate with others who are hostile, angry, or upset. It is important to remember how to communicate effectively. Here are some tips to help you keep cool during communication.

Communicating with Residents

♦ Address residents by titles or names they prefer, not by pet names such as Sweetie, Honey, Grandma, or Gramps.

♦ Keep your conversations "client-centered." Try to keep residents talking about themselves, rather than you talking about yourself.

♦ Be respectful and kind when speaking with all residents. Speak to the elderly as adults, even if they are confused.

♦ Include residents in your conversation; avoid talking to coworkers as though the resident was not present.

♦ Remember that your body language is also a form of communication. Make your nonverbal communication match your words.

♦ Listen carefully when residents speak to you, giving them your full attention.

- Tell a visually impaired resident that you are in the room, then gently touch the resident to let him know that you are near.

- Stand in front of residents with hearing problems when you speak so they can see your mouth and more easily read your lips.

Communicating with Family and Friends of Residents

- Be helpful, friendly, and positive when communicating with visitors.

- Remember to maintain the resident's confidentiality. Avoid discussing confidential information about the resident with visitors.

- Listen attentively to concerns or criticisms of care; avoid becoming defensive.

- Refer questions about medications, diagnosis, and treatment to the supervising nurse.

- Be courteous and kind to visitors, treating them as guests in the facility.

- Take action on a visitor's complaint or concern. If you are unable to do this, pass the complaint or concern along to the appropriate person.

Communicating with Coworkers

♦ Listen carefully when you are given assignments or requested to perform tasks.

♦ Take notes to help you remember your priorities and responsibilities.

♦ Give complete information when you report to your supervising nurse.

♦ Realize that sometimes coworkers need a listening ear, and allow them to vent their feelings about their work.

♦ Go to the co-worker you have a conflict with and discuss it with him or her. Avoid discussing the conflict with other people instead.

6 BREATHING EASY WITH RESPIRATORY CARE

It is easy to become alarmed when a resident is having trouble breathing. The best way to help a resident who is short of breath is to remain calm and reassuring. Then follow these guidelines to assist the resident who has a respiratory problem.

Preventing Respiratory Complications

♦ Elevate the head of the bed for a resident who is short of breath. This will help the resident be able to breathe easier by allowing the lungs to expand better. If a resident is very short of breath, she may need the bed elevated to a sitting position.

♦ Turn bed-bound residents every two hours. This helps prevent mucus from pooling in the lungs and causing pneumonia.

♦ Keep the head of the bed elevated 30 degrees at all times when a resident is receiving a tube feeding. This helps prevent aspiration of the formula, which can cause aspiration pneumonia.

♦ Report any episodes of choking, since aspiration pneumonia can be caused by choking on food, liquid, or vomit.

♦ Encourage residents who are not mobile to take deep breaths and cough from the lungs every two hours to help prevent pooling of mucus in the lungs.

Assisting with Oxygen

♦ Check the resident's ears and head to be sure the mask or cannula strap is not causing pressure areas.

♦ Check the oxygen tubing to be sure it is not kinked or pinched.

♦ Give good oral care to residents receiving oxygen. Oxygen dries out the mouth and nose, so those areas need to be kept moist and clean.

♦ Check the humidifier to be sure that the water is at the correct level and is bubbling.

♦ Be sure that all safety rules for oxygen are followed by residents, staff, and visitors. No smoking or candles should be allowed in a room where a resident is on oxygen therapy. No flammable liquids or electrical equipment that could cause a spark should be used near oxygen.

Caring for Residents with Breathing Problems

♦ Allow time for residents to rest between activities of daily living. Many residents with respiratory illnesses become short of breath while eating, dressing, or bathing. They must rest between those activities to have enough air to accomplish each one.

◆ Encourage residents to do as much as possible for themselves, even though it is tiring for them. Always allow the resident to be as independent as possible.

◆ Encourage residents to drink fluids to help thin mucus and make it easier to cough out. Offer water and other drinks the residents enjoy every two hours. If the resident is on fluid restriction, offer only the approved amounts for your shift.

When a resident has a circulatory problem, the heart, blood vessels, or both may be affected. It is important for you to observe and report any symptoms that could indicate the presence or worsening of a circulatory problem. Here are some guidelines to help you know what to report and how to care for residents with these problems.

♦ Check the blood pressure of a resident with heart disease very carefully. Be sure to report readings that are above 140/90 or below 90/60.

♦ Notice if the resident's feet are cool to touch, a bluish color, or pale. These can all be signs of poor circulation and should be reported to your supervising nurse.

Caring for Residents with Congestive Heart Failure (CHF)

♦ Stay with any resident who complains of chest pain and notify your supervising nurse immediately. Chest pain may be an indication of angina, myocardial infarction (MI), or congestive heart failure (CHF).

♦ Elevate the resident's feet if he or she has congestive heart failure or circulatory problems. When the resident is sitting in a chair, the feet should be elevated on a footstool or pillows to prevent swelling.

♦ Notice increased swelling of the resident's hands or feet. Be aware of moist-sounding coughs and decreased urine output. These symptoms indicate that the resident's body is retaining fluid and increasing the work of the heart. Report any of these findings to your supervising nurse immediately.

Caring for Residents Who Have Had Myocardial Infarctions (MI)

♦ Allow for rest periods during care. The resident may become fatigued or short of breath due to heart damage.

♦ Stay with any resident who complains of chest pain and notify your supervising nurse immediately. Chest pain may be an indication of angina, myocardial infarction (MI), or congestive heart failure (CHF).

♦ Report any irregular or rapid pulse, increased shortness of breath, or cyanosis to your supervising nurse immediately.

♦ Encourage residents to do as much as possible for themselves, while preventing them from overexerting themselves.

Caring for Residents with Artificial Pacemakers

♦ Keep the resident 10 feet away from microwave ovens when they are in use, since they can interfere with the action of some pacemakers.

♦ Notice and report any redness or swelling around the site of the implanted pacemaker.

♦ Take the resident's pulse for a full minute. Report the pulse immediately if it is less than the preset rate of the pacemaker. The resident's chart should contain information about the pacemaker's set rate, which is often set at 60 or 72.

8 MANAGING STROKE CARE

A cerebrovascular accident (CVA), or stroke, occurs when blood flow to the brain is interrupted. It may be caused by a blood clot or a blood vessel rupture in the brain. The part of the brain that does not get oxygenated blood cannot function. Usually one side of the body is weakened or paralyzed by the stroke. This is referred to as the affected side. Residents who have had a stroke have special care needs. Follow these guidelines to master caring for those who have had a stroke.

Assisting with Food and Liquids

♦ Place food in the unaffected side of the resident's mouth when feeding a resident who has had a stroke.

♦ Allow plenty of time for the resident to chew and swallow food before offering the next bite. Be alert to any signs of choking or difficulty swallowing.

♦ Cut food in bite-size pieces, open condiments, and butter bread for the resident who has weakness or paralysis on one side, but is able to feed herself.

♦ Follow the care plan for individual residents. Some may require the use of a thickening agent in liquids and may need to take liquids from a spoon rather than from a cup or straw.

Assisting with Mobility

♦ Place the wheelchair on the unaffected (strong) side of the resident, when assisting with a transfer from bed to wheelchair. When transferring the resident from the wheelchair to the bed, place the wheelchair so that the resident is transferring toward his unaffected (strong) side.

♦ Dress the affected (weak) limb before dressing the unaffected side. Undress the affected (weak) limb last.

♦ Position the resident in a chair or wheelchair to prevent leaning to the affected (weak) side. Check on her often while she is in a chair or wheelchair.

♦ Assist the resident if he is able to ambulate. Use a gait belt and stand slightly behind the resident on the weak side during ambulation.

Assisting with Communication

♦ Allow time for residents who have had a stroke to speak. The stroke can affect the speech centers of the brain, making speech slow and difficult.

♦ Use appropriate alternative methods for communication if the resident is unable to speak. Picture boards, magic slates, and other devices may be used.

Assisting with Emotional Needs

♦ Allow the resident to express his frustration over his situation. Some residents cry, others become angry. Do not take any expression of emotion as a personal attack on you.

♦ Celebrate all accomplishments, however small, to encourage residents who have had a stroke.

♦ Be kind, considerate, and caring when you interact with residents who have had a stroke.

9 DEALING WITH DISORIENTATION AND CONFUSION

When a resident is confused or disoriented to time, place, and/or person, you can use many strategies to help the resident cope with the anxiety and fear that can arise from this condition. Here are some guidelines and strategies to help patients who are confused or disruptive.

Keeping the Environment Calm

♦ Stay calm and in control. Keep the environment calm as well, to avoid over-stimulating the resident.

♦ Keep to a scheduled routine. Residents often find security in a daily routine, without unexpected disruptions.

♦ Remove the resident from a situation that is causing overwhelming anxiety. Take the resident to a quiet, calm environment to help calm him or her.

♦ Ensure safety for residents who are confused or disoriented. These residents are most at risk for accidents and injuries because they do not recognize dangers to themselves.

Communicating with the Disoriented or Confused Resident

♦ Speak slowly, in short and simple sentences. If you sense that speaking to the resident is confusing him or her, wait quietly until the resident is calmer before speaking again.

♦ Use appropriate touch to reassure the resident of your presence and intent.

♦ Approach the resident from the front, rather than the back or side; this will prevent the resident from being threatened by an unexpected presence.

♦ Remind the resident of the appropriate time and place, without contradicting the resident or causing hostility.

♦ Avoid arguing with or scolding a resident; this will only cause embarrassment. Instead, distract the resident and redirect the behavior or conversation.

♦ Reassure residents who are fearful or anxious. Tell them where they are and assure them that they are safe. Validate their feeling as well.

♦ Look for possible causes of increased confusion or anxiety. These can be physical problems as well as emotional triggers.

Communicating with the Resident's Family

♦ Be supportive and helpful to the family members of residents who are disoriented and confused. Allow them to talk about their feelings and responses when they see a loved one in this situation.

Diabetes mellitus occurs when the resident's body cannot produce and use insulin properly. The resident's blood sugar is elevated when insulin is not present to change sugar to energy. Oral medications and insulin injections are used to treat diabetes mellitus. Diabetic residents may have hypoglycemic (low blood sugar) reactions to the medication or they may have hyperglycemia (high blood sugar) if the medications are not effective. Several other complications can occur as a result of diabetes. Follow these guidelines to help defeat diabetic complications.

Reporting Signs of Blood Sugar Imbalance

♦ Watch for cold, clammy, pale skin; shallow respirations; a rapid, thready pulse, and nervousness or shaking. Report these signs of hypoglycemia to your supervising nurse immediately.

♦ Watch for hot, dry, flushed skin; slow, deep respirations; a fruity breath odor; nausea, and sluggishness. Report these signs of hyperglycemia to your supervising nurse immediately.

Assisting with Food and Fluids

♦ Encourage residents with diabetes to eat all the food served on their trays. Report any uneaten food according to the policy at your facility.

- ♦ Serve snacks on time and encourage the resident to eat the complete snack. Report any uneaten snacks according to facility policy.

- ♦ Discourage friends and family members from bringing food to the resident with diabetes. Suggest nonfood items as treats instead.

Assisting with Foot Care

- ♦ Wash, dry, and examine the resident's feet daily. Report any signs of discoloration or injury.

- ♦ Report any injury immediately, even if it is very slight.

- ♦ Always place well-fitting shoes and socks on the resident's feet before she ambulates to prevent accidental injury to the toes or feet.

- ♦ Inspect toenails for length and redness. Notify your supervising nurse if the resident needs his toenails trimmed or has ingrown toenails.

- ♦ Make sure that there are no holes in the resident's socks and no areas of the shoes that rub on the foot. Anything that can cause a sore or blister can lead to serious infection for a resident with diabetes.

Protecting Residents from Injury

♦ Inspect the resident's skin during bathing and pericare. Report any reddened or open areas to your supervising nurse immediately.

♦ Assist residents with water temperatures to prevent burns, since diabetes can cause loss of sensation in the extremities.

♦ Assist residents with ambulation and activities, if needed, since diabetes can affect vision.

♦ Encourage the resident to be active. Exercise helps increase circulation, stimulates appetite, and aids digestion.

11 OVERCOMING PROBLEMS IN OBSERVING, REPORTING, AND RECORDING

As a certified nursing assistant, you are in the position to observe a great deal about the residents you care for. Your observations are important and must be reported to the appropriate person. Then the resident's condition and response to care can be fully evaluated. Some tips to use when observing residents and reporting your observations are:

Gathering Objective Data

♦ Collect information about residents by making objective observations. You will make those observations using your senses of sight, touch, hearing, and smell.

♦ Look for any unusual appearance of the resident or the resident's skin. Notice drainage from wounds and the color of secretions.

♦ Listen for unusual sounds such as slurred speech, wheezing, coughing, or moaning.

♦ Notice unusual odors on the resident's breath, from a wound, in urine, or in stool.

♦ Feel for anything unusual such as swelling, fever, or irregular pulse.

Gathering Subjective Data

♦ Collect information about residents by listening to what residents tells you about how they are feeling. This information cannot be objectively observed, so you must rely on the information given to you by the resident.

♦ Listen for complaints of pain or headache.

♦ Listen for complaints of nausea.

♦ Listen for complaints of dizziness.

♦ Listen for feelings of sadness, depression, or worthlessness.

♦ Look for changes in facial expression and non-verbal communication.

♦ Ask questions to be sure you understand the subjective information the resident is telling you.

Reporting Your Observations

♦ Report all abnormal findings to your supervising nurse.

♦ Keep notes to yourself, so you can give accurate and complete information when you report to your supervising nurse.

♦ Be objective when you report. Give factual information, not vague reports or your opinions.

♦ Report subtle changes in the resident's behavior. If a resident "just doesn't seem himself," let your supervising nurse know about the change.

♦ Use words with clear meanings when you report. Instead of saying a resident "feels bad," say that the resident complains of nausea.

Recording Your Observations

♦ Record, or chart, your factual observations in the resident's chart according to the policy at your facility.

♦ Include the date and time of the observation.

♦ Record only on a page that contains information identifying the resident.

♦ Record in the correct section of the chart. Be sure you have the right resident's chart before you begin to write.

♦ Draw a line through any errors and note them as such. Do not erase or use correction fluid on a chart.

♦ Write in chronological order, leaving no empty lines or spaces.

♦ Sign your entry with your signature and title.

♦ Use correct grammar, spelling, and standard abbreviations.

12 GIVING ATTENTION TO ABNORMAL FINDINGS

Your skills of observation are very important in providing the best care possible for your residents. You will have the most contact with residents and will be the first to notice anything unusual. Here are some tips on how to sharpen your skills of observation.

Observing the Skin

♦ Observe for abnormal colors such as redness, cyanosis, bruising, or paleness.

♦ Observe for broken areas such as cracks, rash, skin tears, sores, or wounds.

♦ Feel skin for temperature. Notice any area that is warmer or cooler than the rest of the skin.

♦ Check skin folds, under arms, and in the groin area to observe for abnormal skin condition.

Observing the Bones, Muscles, and Joints

♦ Notice any decrease in range of motion in joints.

♦ Observe residents for difficulty bearing weight or moving a limb.

♦ Observe residents' gait for unevenness, such as a limp or the favoring of one leg or foot.

♦ Notice any stiffness in a limb or a resident's inability to use a limb.

Observing the Heart and Circulation

♦ Notice any differences in pulses on the left and right side of the body.

♦ Listen and feel for an irregular heartbeat; feel for a weak, thready, or bounding pulse.

♦ Notice any differences in temperature in one limb compared to the other limb.

♦ Observe for swelling in the feet and ankles.

♦ Observe for blood pressure readings above 140/90 or below 90/60.

♦ Note a pulse above 90 or below 60.

Observing Respirations

♦ Listen for abnormal respiratory sounds such as wheezes, gurgles, or crackles.

♦ Note the rhythm and depth of respirations.

♦ Note a respiratory rate above 20 or below 16.

♦ Observe residents for shortness of breath during activity and at rest.

♦ Observe the flow rate of oxygen if it is in use.

Observing Elimination

♦ Notice how frequently residents have bowel movements. Tell your supervising nurse if a resident has gone two days (48 hours) without having a bowel movement.

♦ Notice black, green, tarry, or bloody stools.

♦ Observe stool for consistency; note diarrhea, loose, or pasty stools. Residents who are tube fed normally have pasty stools.

♦ Notice any abnormal odors from the bowel movement.

♦ Observe urine for color: note brown, tea-colored, dark amber, or orange urine.

♦ Notice any sediment or mucus in the urine.

♦ Observe the amount of urine each time a resident voids. Voids of less than 200 mL at a time may indicate a urinary tract infection or incomplete emptying of the bladder.

Observing Neurological Status

♦ Notice any changes in a resident's usual awareness of person, place, and time.

♦ Notice any change in a resident's usual behavior, such as combativeness, confusion, or despair.

- Notice any change in the resident's usual level of awareness, such as being difficult to arouse or sleeping a great deal more than usual.

- Notice any changes in the resident's speech, such as slurring or the incorrect use of words.

Reporting Abnormals

- Report all abnormal findings to your supervising nurse immediately.

- Give thorough, accurate, and objective information when reporting abnormal findings.

- Report abnormal findings to the appropriate person if your supervising nurse is not available.

In order for long-term care facilities to retain their licenses to operate, the facility is inspected periodically by a survey team. Any problems found during the inspection are noted as deficiencies. The long-term care facility must develop and implement a plan to correct these problems. As a Certified Nursing Assistant, you have a big role in keeping your facility ready for a survey team to visit. Facilities that also admit residents funded by Medicare may have a separate inspection by Medicare officials. Here are some tips to help you survive the survey when your facility is inspected.

Using Standard Precautions

♦ Always practice standard precautions. Wear gloves when you give direct care to any resident.

♦ Remove your gloves before you leave a resident's room. Do not wear gloves into the hall or wear the same gloves in a different resident's room.

♦ Change gloves between caring for residents who are roommates.

♦ Wash your hands before putting on gloves and after removing gloves.

♦ Wash your hands when you leave a resident's room and before touching another resident.

Keeping Equipment and Supplies Ready

♦ Keep unused equipment, extra wheelchairs, and other items out of hallways. These items should be stored in appropriate storage areas.

♦ Keep clean linens covered while on the linen cart.

♦ Place soiled linens in the appropriate container and immediately replace the lid. If the container is too full for the lid to fit on tightly, take the linen container to the laundry area to be emptied and bring back an empty container.

♦ Take only the amount of linen you need into a resident's room; do not bring linen out of a resident's room and return it to the linen cart.

♦ Clean and disinfect any equipment that is taken from room to room according to facility policy.

Performing Your Duties

♦ Care for all residents as you would when the survey team is not present.

♦ Provide privacy for residents at all times; be sure residents are clothed going to and from the shower or tub.

♦ Respond to resident's questions and requests courteously and quickly.

♦ Assist with meals as usual; ensure that food is served at the correct temperature.

- Keep all food in the appropriate location; food should not be open and left at the resident's bedside.

- Use good body mechanics and safe transfer practices.

- Place call lights within reach of residents at all times.

- Answer call lights promptly.

- Stay calm and kind. You may be aware of tension among staff during a survey team's visit, but do not become tense in response.

- Give good care to all residents at all times. This will help your facility do well during the inspection.

NOTES